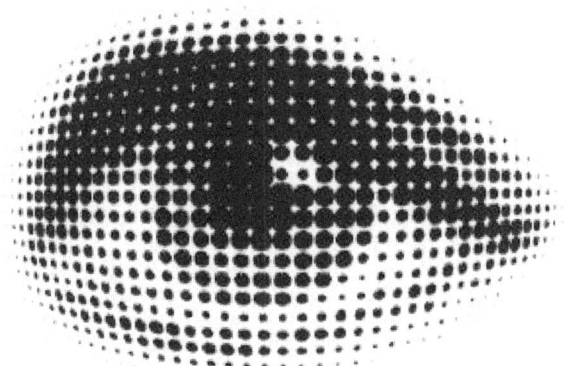

speak

Larry Dillingham

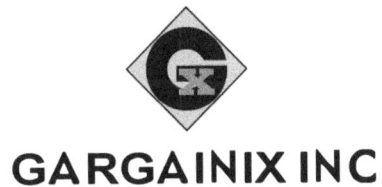

Eye Speak

Copyright © 2019 by Gargainix Inc (Larry Dillingham). All rights reserved.

No part of this publication may be reproduced, stored in a retrieval system or transmitted in any way by any means, electronic, mechanical photocopy, recording or otherwise without the prior permission of the author except as provided by USA copyright law.

This book is designed to provide accurate and authoritative information with regard t o the subject matter covered. This information is given with the understanding that neither the author nor Gargainix Inc is engaged in rendering legal, professional advice. Since the details of your situation are fact dependent, you should additionally seek the services of a competent professional.

The opinions expressed by the author are not necessarily those of Gargainix Inc.

Published by Gargainix Inc
P.O. Box 853 | Holbrook, New York 11741 USA
1.631.954.1204 | www.gargainix.com

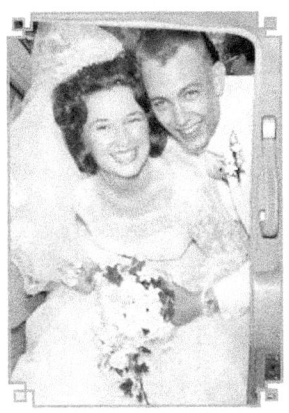

Individuals living with the condition called Locked-in Syndrome can now write messages and communicate with their family and friends, lawyers and business partners. Using this book with a partner, an individual can write a message or letter with only the ability to blink. They accomplish this by working through the book to select one letter at a time until they have completed the intended message. It's that simple!

How to use:

1. Sit facing your partner with extra paper by your side to write the message.
2. Open the book so that you can see the back of the cards known as the instruction side.
3. Take a minute to get accustomed to how your partner blinks. It will be important that you count correctly.
4. Start with page 1, show them the page, and count the number of times they blink. Explain that if they make a mistake and want to return to the previous page, they can do this by not blinking. If you decide to not use control words, then start with page 2.
5. Follow the directions on the instruction side of the card.
6. Keep repeating this process until your partner is finished with their message.

1

1 BLINK

A B C D E F G H
I J K L M N O P
Q R S T U V W
X Y Z
0 1 2 3 4 5 6 7 8 9

2 BLINKS

[space]
[end of sentence]
[start new letter]
[take a break]

001

1 Blink	Turn to page 2
2 Blinks	Turn to page 33

A B C D E
F G H I J K
L M N O P

1 BLINK

Q R S T U
V W X Y Z
0 1 2 3 4 5 6 7 8 9

2 BLINKS

002

1 Blink	Turn to page 3
2 Blinks	Turn to page 18
NO BLINKS	Go back to page 1

A B C D E F G H

1 BLINK

I J K L M N O P

2 BLINKS

003

1 Blink	Turn to page 4
2 Blinks	Turn to page 11
NO BLINKS	Go back to page 2

A B
C D

1 BLINK

E F
G H

2 BLINKS

004

| 1 Blink | Turn to page 5 |
| 2 Blinks | Turn to page 8 |

| NO BLINKS | Go back to page 3 |

A B

C D

1 BLINK

2 BLINKS

005

1 Blink	Turn to page 6
2 Blinks	Turn to page 7
NO BLINKS	Go back to page 4

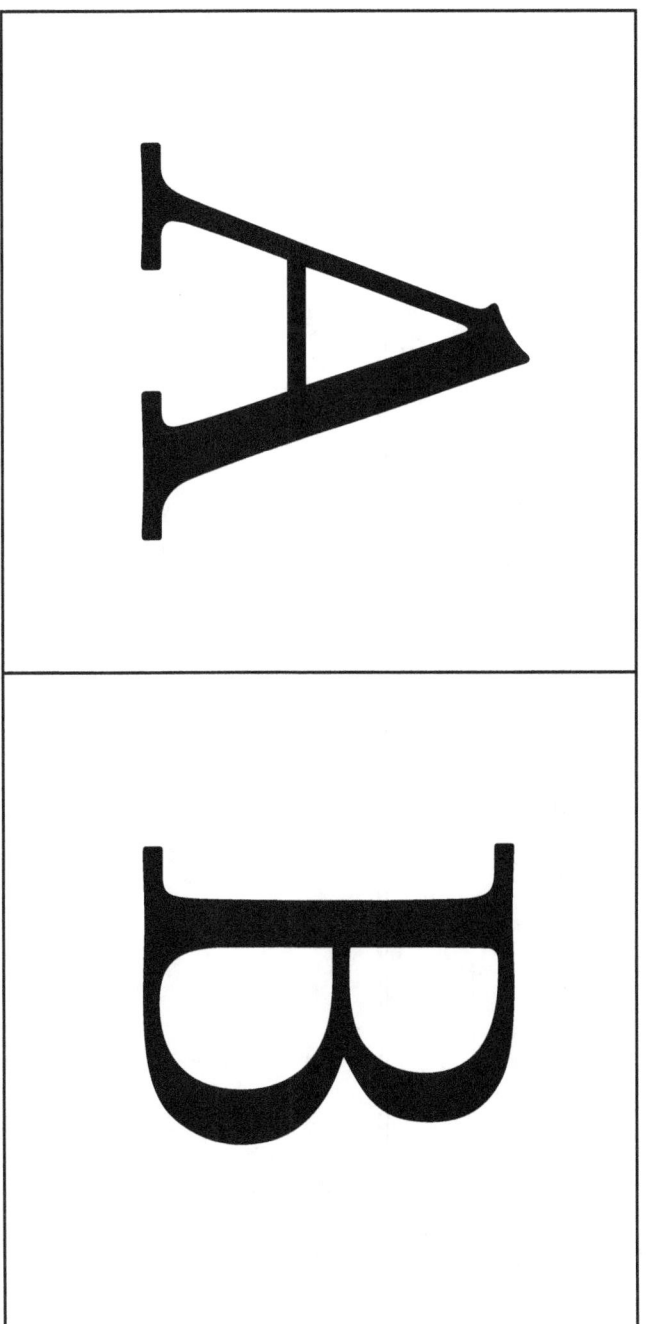

1 BLINK

2 BLINKS

006

1 Blink	Write the letter A and turn to page 1
2 Blinks	Write the letter B and turn to page 1
NO BLINKS	Go back to page 5

Ω

1 BLINK

D

2 BLINKS

007

1 Blink	Write the letter C and turn to page 1
2 Blinks	Write the letter D and turn to page 1
NO BLINKS	Go back to page 5

E F

1 BLINK

G H

2 BLINKS

008

1 Blink	Turn to page 9
2 Blinks	Turn to page 10
NO BLINKS	Go back to page 4

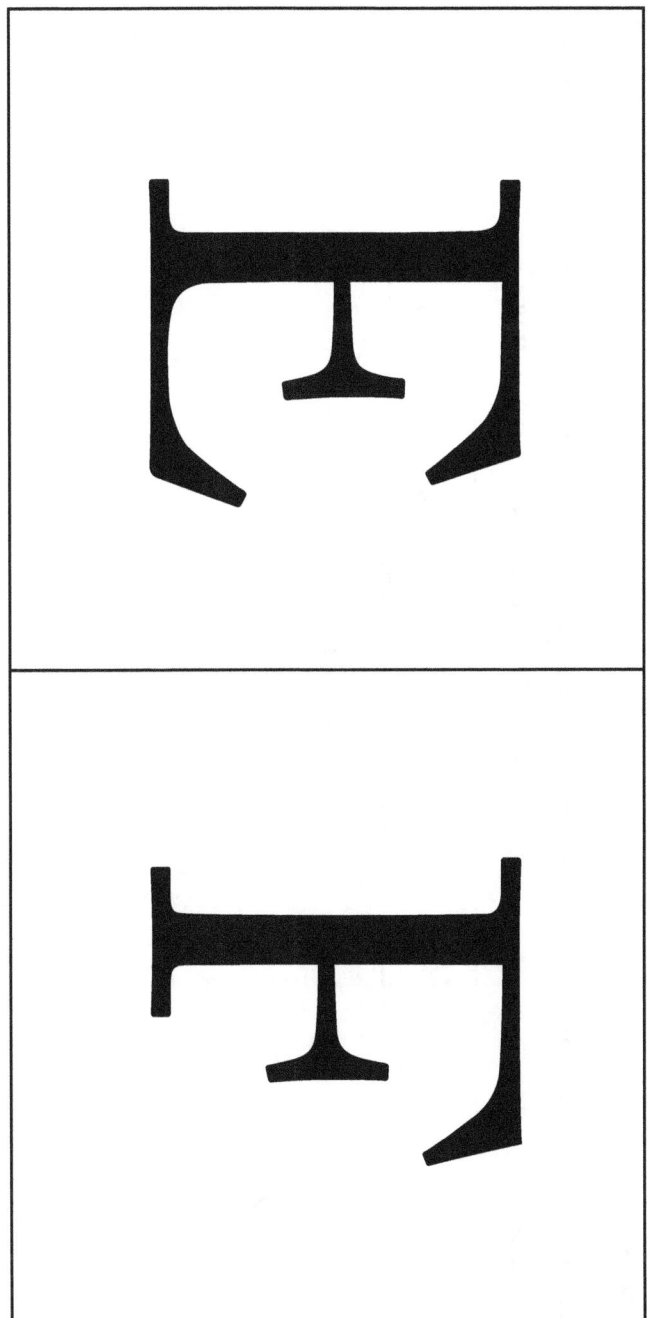

1 BLINK

2 BLINKS

009

1 Blink	Write the letter E and turn to page 1
2 Blinks	Write the letter F and turn to page 1
NO BLINKS	Go back to page 8

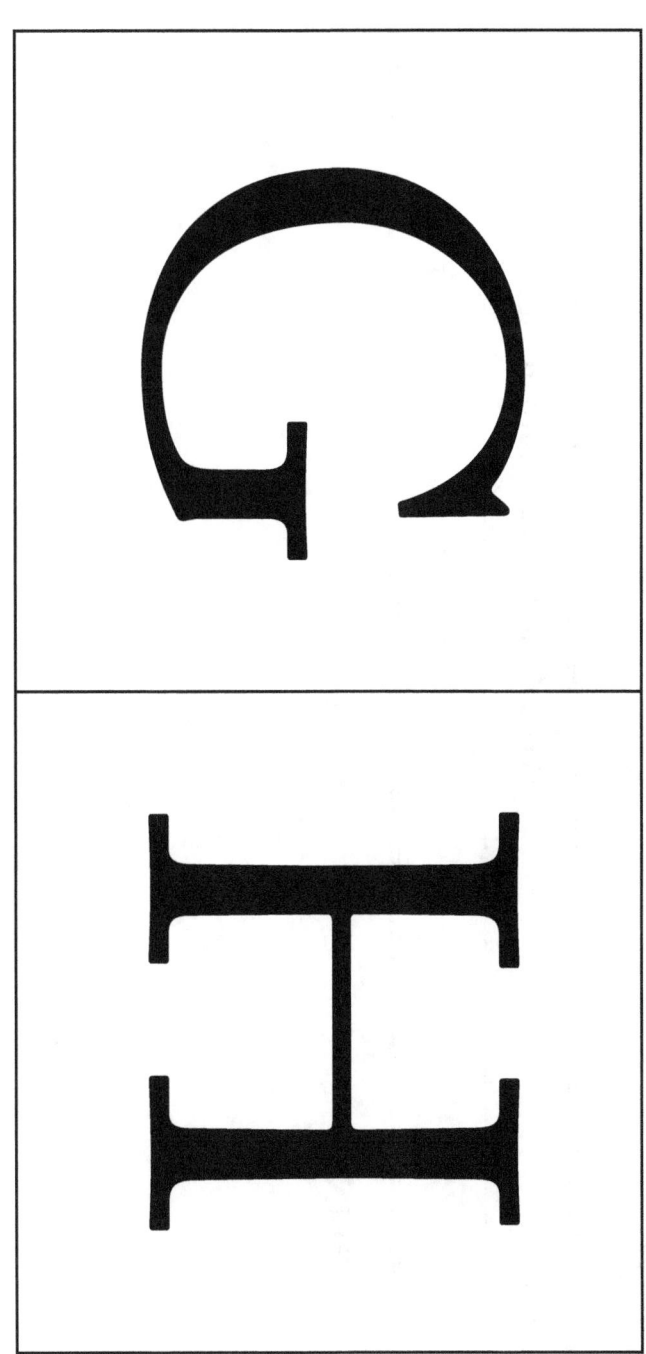

01

1 BLINK

2 BLINKS

010

1 Blink	Write the letter G and turn to page 1
2 Blinks	Write the letter H and turn to page 1

NO BLINKS — Go back to page 8

I J
K L

1 BLINK

M N
O P

2 BLINKS

011

1 Blink	Turn to page 12
2 Blinks	Turn to page 15
NO BLINKS	Go back to page 3

IJ

1 BLINK

KL

2 BLINKS

012

1 Blink	Turn to page 13
2 Blinks	Turn to page 14
NO BLINKS	Go back to page 11

1 BLINK

2 BLINKS

013

1 Blink	Write the letter I and turn to page 1
2 Blinks	Write the letter J and turn to page 1
NO BLINKS	Go back to page 12

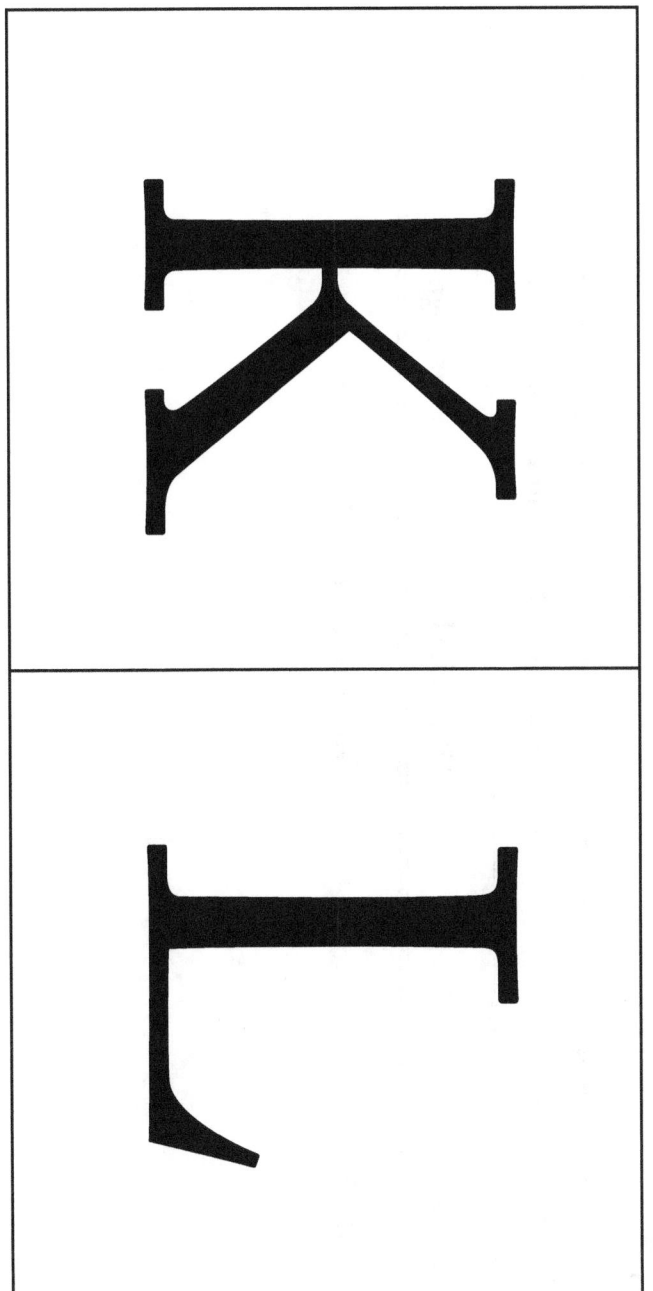

1 BLINK

2 BLINKS

014

1 Blink	Write the letter K and turn to page 1
2 Blinks	Write the letter L and turn to page 1
NO BLINKS	Go back to page 12

15

1 BLINK

2 BLINKS

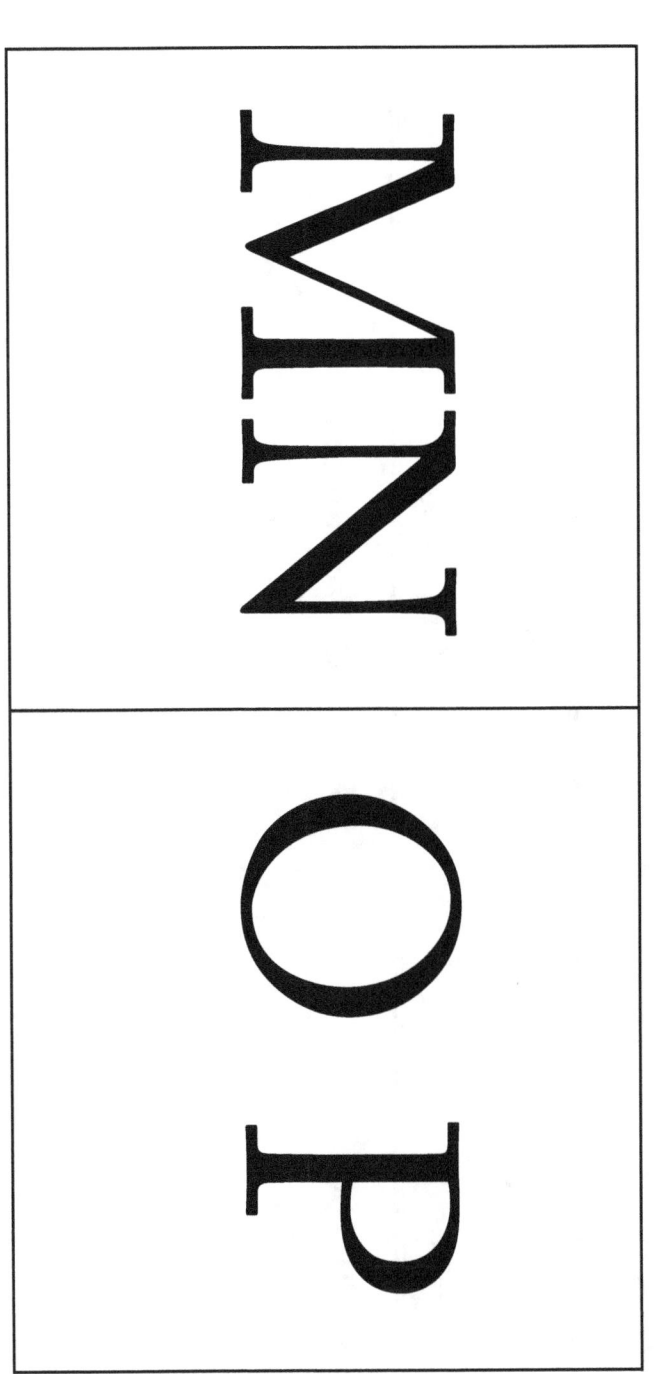

015

1 Blink	Turn to page 16
2 Blinks	Turn to page 17
NO BLINKS	Go back to page 11

M

1 BLINK

N

2 BLINKS

016

1 Blink	Write the letter M and turn to page 1
2 Blinks	Write the letter N and turn to page 1
NO BLINKS	Go back to page 15

17

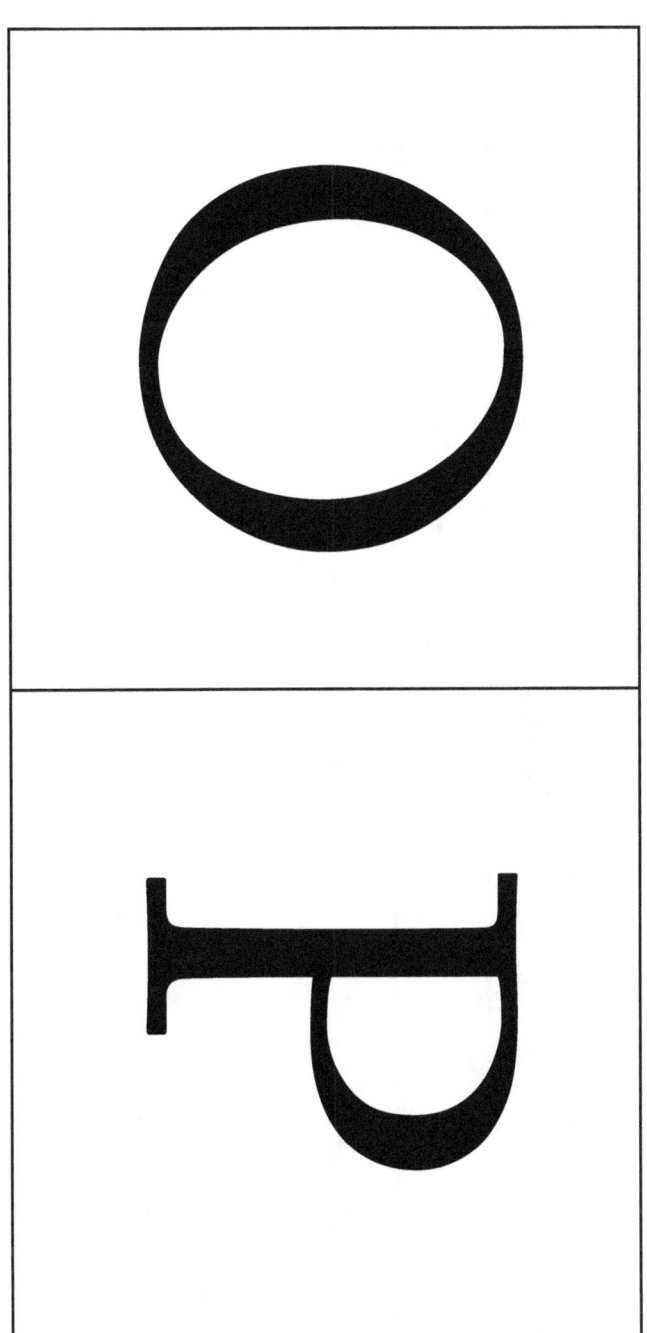

1 BLINK

2 BLINKS

017

1 Blink	Write the letter O and turn to page 1
2 Blinks	Write the letter P and turn to page 1
NO BLINKS	Go back to page 15

1 BLINK

2 BLINKS

QRS
TUV
WX

YZ
01234
56789

018

1 Blink	Turn to page 19
2 Blinks	Turn to page 26
NO BLINKS	Go back to page 2

Q R S T

1 BLINK

U V W X

2 BLINKS

019

1 Blink	Turn to page 20
2 Blinks	Turn to page 23
NO BLINKS	Go back to page 18

20

Q R
S T

1 BLINK

2 BLINKS

020

1 Blink	Turn to page 21
2 Blinks	Turn to page 22
NO BLINKS	Go back to page 19

21

1 BLINK

2 BLINKS

021

1 Blink — Write the letter Q and turn to page 1

2 Blinks — Write the letter R and turn to page 1

NO BLINKS — Go back to page 20

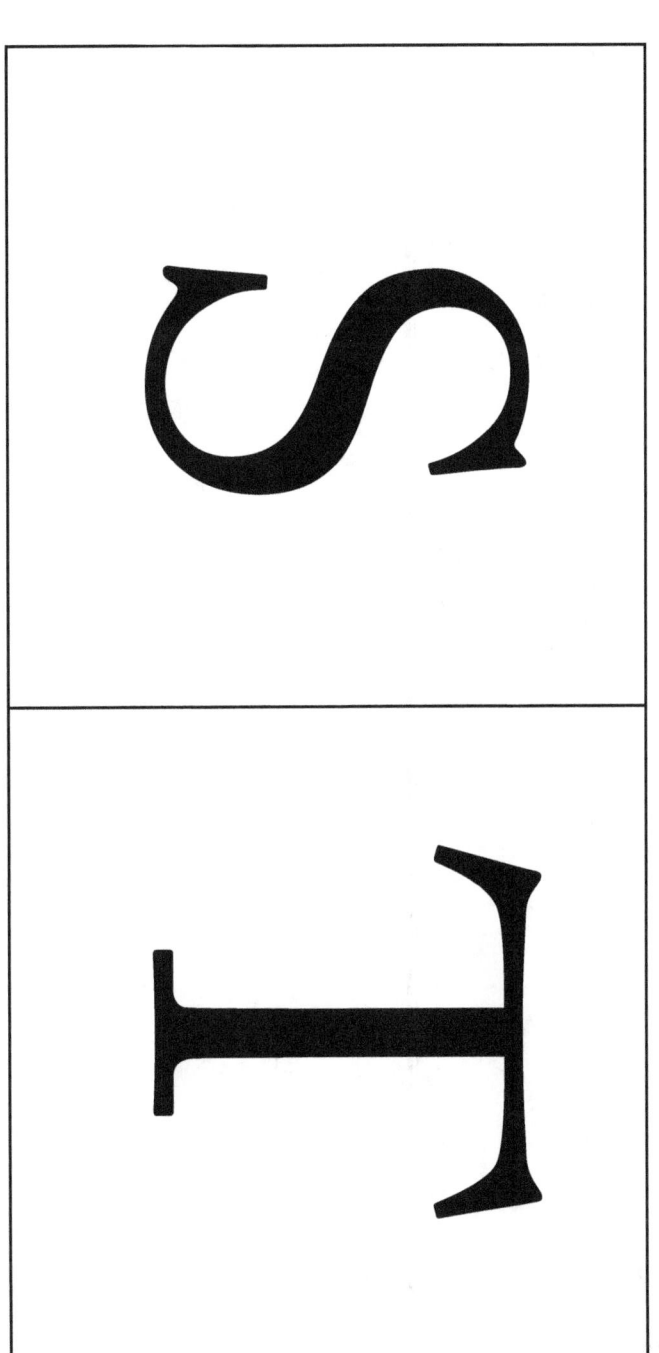

1 BLINK

2 BLINKS

22

022

1 Blink | Write the letter S and turn to page 1

2 Blinks | Write the letter T and turn to page 1

NO BLINKS | Go back to page 20

23

U V

1 BLINK

W X

2 BLINKS

023

1 Blink	Turn to page 24
2 Blinks	Turn to page 25
NO BLINKS	Go back to page 19

U

1 BLINK

A

2 BLINKS

024

1 Blink	Write the letter U and turn to page 1
2 Blinks	Write the letter V and turn to page 1

NO BLINKS — Go back to page 23

25

W	X
1 BLINK	2 BLINKS

025

1 Blink	Write the letter W and turn to page 1
2 Blinks	Write the letter X and turn to page 1

NO BLINKS — Go back to page 23

1 BLINK	2 BLINKS
Y Z 0 1 2 3	4 5 6 7 8 9

026

1 Blink	Turn to page 27
2 Blinks	Turn to page 30
NO BLINKS	Go back to page 18

Y Z 0

1 BLINK

1 2 3

2 BLINKS

027

| 1 Blink | Turn to page 28 |
| 2 Blinks | Turn to page 29 |

| NO BLINKS | Go back to page 26 |

Y	Z	O
1 BLINK	2 BLINKS	3 BLINK

028

1 Blink	Write the letter Y and turn to page 1
2 Blinks	Write the letter Z and turn to page 1
3 Blinks	Write the number 0 and turn to page 1
NO BLINKS	Go back to page 27

1

1 BLINK

2

2 BLINKS

3

3 BLINKS

029

1 Blink	Write the number 1 and turn to page 1
2 Blinks	Write the number 2 and turn to page 1
3 Blinks	Write the number 3 and turn to page 1
NO BLINKS	Go back to page 27

30

4 5 6	7 8 9
1 BLINK	2 BLINKS

030

1 Blink	Turn to page 31
2 Blinks	Turn to page 32
NO BLINKS	Go back to page 26

31

4	1 BLINK
5	2 BLINKS
6	3 BLINKS

031

1 Blink	Write the number 4 and turn to page 1
2 Blinks	Write the number 5 and turn to page 1
3 Blinks	Write the number 6 and turn to page 1
NO BLINKS	Go back to page 30

32

7	1 BLINK
8	2 BLINKS
9	3 BLINKS

032

1 Blink	Write the number 7 and turn to page 1
2 Blinks	Write the number 8 and turn to page 1
3 Blinks	Write the number 9 and turn to page 1
NO BLINKS	Go back to page 30

SPACE

1 BLINK

[end of sentence]
[start new letter]
[take a break]

2 BLINKS

033

1 Blink	Leave a space and turn to page 1
2 Blinks	Turn to page 34
NO BLINKS	Go back to page 1

1 BLINK	2 BLINKS	3 BLINKS
END OF SENTENCE	START NEW LETTER	TAKE A BREAK

034

1 Blink — Write a " . " and leave a space and turn to page 1

2 Blinks — Start a new letter and turn to page 1

3 Blinks — Take a break and turn to page 1

NO BLINKS — Go back to page 33

Being trapped in a "Locked-In" State is no joking matter! For this reason, I will always strive to minimize the cost to keep this available on the online market.

My hope is that you are able to communicate with your loved one, and fulfill my original purpose when I created this so many years ago.

I unfortunate didn't get this completed before my father passed. If even one person can benefit from my efforts, I'd consider that a major success!

If you'd like to make a donation to future projects... any amount is appreciated.

To make donations via Check:
(Please make checks to: Larry Dillingham)

Send them to:
Gargainix Inc
c/o Larry Dillingham
P.O. Box 853
Holbrook, NY 11741

To send a donation via Paypal:
Please use : **larrydillingham@gargainix.com**

Do you have a comment or suggestion?
I'd love to hear what you think about this workbook, and your story...
Send messages to: **larrydillingham@gargainix.com**

www.ingramcontent.com/pod-product-compliance
Lightning Source LLC
Chambersburg PA
CBHW070439180526
45158CB00019B/1768